W9-CTP-051

Pregnant females: First trimester, ≤ 500,000 IU/24 hours; second trimester, 10,000 to 25,000 IU/24 hours; third trimester, 5,000 to 15,000 IU/24 hours

Clot retraction
50%

Coccidioidomycosis antibody, serum
Normal titer < 1:2

Cold agglutinins, serum
Normal titer < 1:16

Complement, serum
Total: 41 to 90 hemolytic units
CI esterase inhibitor: 16 to 33 mg/dl
C3: Males, 88 to 252 mg/dl; females, 88 to 206 mg/dl
C4: Males, 12 to 72 mg/dl; females, 13 to 75 mg/dl

Complement, synovial fluid
10 mg protein/dl: 3.7 to 33.7 units/ml
20 mg protein/dl: 7.7 to 37.7 units/ml

Copper, urine
15 to 60 mcg/24 hours

Copper reduction test, urine
Negative

Coproporphyrin, urine
Men: 0 to 96 mcg/24 hours
Women: 1 to 57 mcg/24 hours

Cortisol, plasma
Morning: 7 to 28 mcg/dl
Afternoon: 2 to 18 mcg/dl

Cortisol, free, urine
24 to 108 mcg/24 hours

Creatine phosphokinase
Total: Men, 23 to 99 units/liter; women, 15 to 57 units/liter
CPK-BB: None
CPK-MB: 0 to 7 IU/liter
CPK-MM: 5 to 70 IU/liter

Creatine, serum
Males: 0.2 to 0.6 mg/dl
Females: 0.6 to 1 mg/dl

Creatinine, amniotic fluid
> 2 mg/100 ml in mature fetus

Creatinine clearance
Men (age 20): 90 ml/minute/1.73 m²
Women (age 20): 84 ml/minute/1.73 m²
For older patients, concentrations normally decrease by 6 ml/minute/decade.

Creatinine, serum
Males: 0.8 to 1.2 mg/dl
Females: 0.6 to 0.9 mg/dl

Creatinine, urine
Men: 1 to 1.9 g/24 hours
Women: 0.8 to 1.7 g/24 hours

Cryoglobulins, serum
Negative

Cryptococcosis antigen, serum
Negative

Cyclic adenosine monophosphate, urine
Parathyroid hormone infusion: 3.6 to 4 μmoles increase

D

Delta-aminolevulinic acid, urine
1.5 to 7.5 mg/dl/24 hours

D-xylose absorption
Blood: Children, 730 mg/dl in 1 hour; adults, 25 to 40 mg/dl in 2 hours
Urine: Children, 16% to 33% excreted in 5 hours; adults, > 3.5 g excreted in 5 hours

E

Erythrocyte sedimentation rate
Males: 0 to 10 mm/hour
Females: 0 to 20 mm/hour

Esophageal acidity
pH > 5.0

Estriol, amniotic fluid
16 to 20 weeks: 25.7 ng/ml
Term: < 1,000 ng/ml

Estrogens, serum
Menstruating females: day 1 to 10, 24 to 68 pg/ml; day 11 to 20, 50 to 186 pg/ml; day 21 to 30, 73 to 149 pg/ml
Males: 12 to 34 pg/ml

Estrogens, total urine
Menstruating females: follicular phase, 5 to 25 mcg/24 hours; ovulatory phase, 24 to 100 mcg/24 hours; luteal phase, 12 to 80 mcg/24 hours
Postmenopausal females: < 10 mcg/24 hours
Males: 4 to 25 mcg/24 hours

Euglobulin lysis time
≥ 2 hours

F

Factor II assay
225 to 290 units/ml

Factor V assay
50% to 150% of control

Factor VII assay
65% to 135% of control

Factor VIII assay
55% to 145% of control

Factor IX assay
60% to 140% of control

Factor X assay
45% to 155% of control

Factor XI assay
65% to 135% of control

Factor XII assay
50% to 150% of control

Ferritin, serum
Men: 20 to 300 ng/ml
Women: 20 to 120 ng/ml

Fibrin split products
Screening assay: < 10 mcg/ml
Quantitative assay: < 3 mcg/ml

Fibrinogen, peritoneal fluid
0.3% to 4.5% of total protein

Fibrinogen, plasma
195 to 365 mg/dl

Fibrinogen, pleural fluid
Transudate: Absent
Exudate: Present

Fibrinogen, synovial fluid
None

Fluorescent treponemal absorption, serum
Negative

Folic acid, serum
2 to 14 ng/ml

Follicle-stimulating hormone, serum
Menstruating females: Follicular phase, 5 to 20 mIU/ml; ovulatory phase, 15 to 30 mIU/ml; luteal phase, 5 to 15 mIU/ml
Menopausal females: 5 to 100 mIU/ml
Males: 5 to 20 mIU/ml

Free fatty acids, plasma
0.3 to 1.0 mEq/liter

Free thyroxine, serum
0.8 to 3.3 ng/dl

Free triiodothyronine
0.2 to 0.6 ng/dl

G

Gamma glutamyl transferase
Males: 6 to 37 units/liter
Females: < age 45, 5 to 27 units/liter; > age 45, 6 to 37 units/liter

Gastric acid stimulation
Males: 18 to 28 mEq/hour
Females: 11 to 21 mEq/hour

Gastric secretion, basal
Males: 1 to 5 mEq/hour
Females: 0.2 to 3.8 mEq/hour

Gastrin, serum
< 300 pg/ml

Globulin, peritoneal fluid
30% to 45% of total protein

Globulin, serum
Alpha₁: 0.1 to 0.4 g/dl
Alpha₂: 0.5 to 1 g/dl
Beta: 0.7 to 1.2 g/dl
Gamma: 0.5 to 1.6 g/dl

Glucose, amniotic fluid
< 45 mg/100 ml

Glucose, cerebrospinal fluid
50 to 80 mg/100 ml

Glucose, fasting, plasma
70 to 100 mg/dl

Glucose, plasma, oral tolerance
Peak at 160 to 180 mg/dl, 30 to 60 minutes after challenge dose

Glucose, plasma, 2-hour postprandial
< 145 mg/dl

Glucose, urine
Negative

Growth hormone, serum
Men: 0 to 5 ng/ml
Women: 0 to 10 ng/ml

Growth hormone stimulation
Men: Increases to ≥ 10 ng/ml
Women: Increases to ≥ 15 ng/ml

Growth hormone suppression
0 to 3 ng/ml after 30 minutes to 2 hours

H

Haptoglobin, serum
38 to 270 mg/dl

Heinz bodies
Negative

(continued inside back cover)

HEALTH ASSESSMENT HANDBOOK

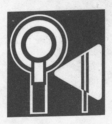

Springhouse Corporation
Springhouse, Pennsylvania

Developmental Editor   Regina Daley Ford
Designer   Lynn Foulk
Copy Supervisor   David Moreau

Adapted from *Assessment* (Nurse's Reference Library®), Copyright 1983, 1982 by Springhouse Corporation. Editorial Director—Diana Odell Potter, Clinical Director—Minnie Bowen Rose, RN, BSN, MEd.

Nursing85 Books™